SWEAT.
IS FAT.
CRYING.

PERSONAL CONTACT DETAILS

NAME	
ADDRESS	
TEL	
EMAIL	

EMERGENCY CONTACT DETAILS

NAME	
TEL	
EMAIL	

ASSESSMENT

(subtract age from 220)

DOB / AGE		HEIGHT		MAX HR	

DATE					
RESTING HEART RATE (BPM)					
BLOOD PRESSURE (MMHG)					
BODY MASS INDEX (BMI)					
BODY WEIGHT					
BODY COMPOSITION (%)					
Fat					
Visceral Fat					
Muscle					
BODY MEASUREMENTS (MM)					
Chest					
Upper Arms					
Thighs					
Waist					
Hips					
Waist / Hip Ratio					
SKIN FOLD MEASUREMENTS (MM)					
Bicep					
Tricep					
Subscapular					
Supra Iliac					
Total mm					
Body Fat %					

1-REP MAX (1RM)

DATE					
1RM					
Bicep Curl					
Back Squat					
Bent Over Row					
Calf Raise					
Chest Press					
Deadlift					
Hip Extension					
Hip Flexion					
Lat Pull Down					
Leg Adduction					
Leg Curl					
Leg Extension					
Leg Press					
Low Row					
Military Press					
Overhead Press					
Power Clean					
Seated Row					
Shoulder Press					
Smith Machine Squat					
Split Squat					
Stiff Leg Deadlift					
Tricep Push Down					

DATE:		MON	TUE	WED	THU	FRI	SAT	SUN

SESSION:

WARM UP

CARDIOVASCULAR WORKOUT

WEIGHTS		SET 1		SET 2		SET 3		SET 4		SET 5	
EXERCISE		WEIGHT	REPS	WEIGHT	REPS	WEIGHT	REPS	WEIGHT	REPS	WEIGHT	REPS

NOTES

<table>
<tr><td>BREAKFAST</td><td>PROTEIN</td><td>FAT</td><td>CARBS</td><td>KCAL</td></tr>
<tr><td></td><td></td><td></td><td></td><td></td></tr>
<tr><td></td><td></td><td></td><td></td><td></td></tr>
<tr><td></td><td></td><td></td><td></td><td></td></tr>
<tr><td></td><td></td><td></td><td></td><td></td></tr>
</table>

<table>
<tr><td>LUNCH</td><td></td><td></td><td></td><td></td></tr>
<tr><td></td><td></td><td></td><td></td><td></td></tr>
<tr><td></td><td></td><td></td><td></td><td></td></tr>
<tr><td></td><td></td><td></td><td></td><td></td></tr>
<tr><td></td><td></td><td></td><td></td><td></td></tr>
</table>

<table>
<tr><td>DINNER</td><td></td><td></td><td></td><td></td></tr>
<tr><td></td><td></td><td></td><td></td><td></td></tr>
<tr><td></td><td></td><td></td><td></td><td></td></tr>
<tr><td></td><td></td><td></td><td></td><td></td></tr>
<tr><td></td><td></td><td></td><td></td><td></td></tr>
</table>

<table>
<tr><td>SNACKS / DRINKS</td><td></td><td></td><td></td><td></td></tr>
<tr><td></td><td></td><td></td><td></td><td></td></tr>
<tr><td></td><td></td><td></td><td></td><td></td></tr>
<tr><td></td><td></td><td></td><td></td><td></td></tr>
<tr><td></td><td></td><td></td><td></td><td></td></tr>
</table>

	PROTEIN	FAT	CARBS	KCAL
DAILY TOTALS				

NOTES

DATE:		MON	TUE	WED	THU	FRI	SAT	SUN

SESSION:

WARM UP

CARDIOVASCULAR WORKOUT

WEIGHTS		SET 1		SET 2		SET 3		SET 4		SET 5	
EXERCISE		WEIGHT	REPS	WEIGHT	REPS	WEIGHT	REPS	WEIGHT	REPS	WEIGHT	REPS

NOTES

BREAKFAST		PROTEIN	FAT	CARBS	KCAL

LUNCH					

DINNER					

SNACKS / DRINKS					

	PROTEIN	FAT	CARBS	KCAL
DAILY TOTALS				

NOTES

DATE:		MON	TUE	WED	THU	FRI	SAT	SUN

SESSION:

WARM UP

CARDIOVASCULAR WORKOUT

WEIGHTS		SET 1		SET 2		SET 3		SET 4		SET 5	
EXERCISE		WEIGHT	REPS	WEIGHT	REPS	WEIGHT	REPS	WEIGHT	REPS	WEIGHT	REPS

NOTES

BREAKFAST	PROTEIN	FAT	CARBS	KCAL

LUNCH	PROTEIN	FAT	CARBS	KCAL

DINNER	PROTEIN	FAT	CARBS	KCAL

SNACKS / DRINKS	PROTEIN	FAT	CARBS	KCAL

	PROTEIN	FAT	CARBS	KCAL
DAILY TOTALS				

NOTES

DATE:			MON	TUE	WED	THU	FRI	SAT	SUN

SESSION:

WARM UP

CARDIOVASCULAR WORKOUT

WEIGHTS		SET 1		SET 2		SET 3		SET 4		SET 5	
EXERCISE	WEIGHT	REPS	WEIGHT	REPS	WEIGHT	REPS	WEIGHT	REPS	WEIGHT	REPS

NOTES

BREAKFAST			PROTEIN	FAT	CARBS	KCAL

LUNCH						

DINNER						

SNACKS / DRINKS						

	PROTEIN	FAT	CARBS	KCAL
DAILY TOTALS				

NOTES

DATE:		MON	TUE	WED	THU	FRI	SAT	SUN

SESSION:

WARM UP

CARDIOVASCULAR WORKOUT

WEIGHTS		SET 1		SET 2		SET 3		SET 4		SET 5	
EXERCISE		WEIGHT	REPS	WEIGHT	REPS	WEIGHT	REPS	WEIGHT	REPS	WEIGHT	REPS

NOTES

<table>
<tr><td>BREAKFAST</td><td>PROTEIN</td><td>FAT</td><td>CARBS</td><td>KCAL</td></tr>
<tr><td></td><td></td><td></td><td></td><td></td></tr>
<tr><td></td><td></td><td></td><td></td><td></td></tr>
<tr><td></td><td></td><td></td><td></td><td></td></tr>
<tr><td></td><td></td><td></td><td></td><td></td></tr>
<tr><td>LUNCH</td><td></td><td></td><td></td><td></td></tr>
<tr><td></td><td></td><td></td><td></td><td></td></tr>
<tr><td></td><td></td><td></td><td></td><td></td></tr>
<tr><td></td><td></td><td></td><td></td><td></td></tr>
<tr><td></td><td></td><td></td><td></td><td></td></tr>
<tr><td>DINNER</td><td></td><td></td><td></td><td></td></tr>
<tr><td></td><td></td><td></td><td></td><td></td></tr>
<tr><td></td><td></td><td></td><td></td><td></td></tr>
<tr><td></td><td></td><td></td><td></td><td></td></tr>
<tr><td></td><td></td><td></td><td></td><td></td></tr>
<tr><td>SNACKS / DRINKS</td><td></td><td></td><td></td><td></td></tr>
<tr><td></td><td></td><td></td><td></td><td></td></tr>
<tr><td></td><td></td><td></td><td></td><td></td></tr>
<tr><td></td><td></td><td></td><td></td><td></td></tr>
<tr><td></td><td></td><td></td><td></td><td></td></tr>
</table>

	PROTEIN	FAT	CARBS	KCAL
DAILY TOTALS				

NOTES

DATE:		MON	TUE	WED	THU	FRI	SAT	SUN

SESSION:

WARM UP

CARDIOVASCULAR WORKOUT

WEIGHTS		SET 1		SET 2		SET 3		SET 4		SET 5	
EXERCISE		WEIGHT	REPS	WEIGHT	REPS	WEIGHT	REPS	WEIGHT	REPS	WEIGHT	REPS

NOTES

BREAKFAST	PROTEIN	FAT	CARBS	KCAL

LUNCH	PROTEIN	FAT	CARBS	KCAL

DINNER	PROTEIN	FAT	CARBS	KCAL

SNACKS / DRINKS	PROTEIN	FAT	CARBS	KCAL

	PROTEIN	FAT	CARBS	KCAL
DAILY TOTALS				

NOTES

DATE:		MON	TUE	WED	THU	FRI	SAT	SUN

SESSION:

WARM UP

CARDIOVASCULAR WORKOUT

WEIGHTS		SET 1		SET 2		SET 3		SET 4		SET 5	
EXERCISE		WEIGHT	REPS	WEIGHT	REPS	WEIGHT	REPS	WEIGHT	REPS	WEIGHT	REPS

NOTES

BREAKFAST	PROTEIN	FAT	CARBS	KCAL

LUNCH	PROTEIN	FAT	CARBS	KCAL

DINNER	PROTEIN	FAT	CARBS	KCAL

SNACKS / DRINKS	PROTEIN	FAT	CARBS	KCAL

	PROTEIN	FAT	CARBS	KCAL
DAILY TOTALS				

NOTES

<table>
<tr><td>DATE:</td><td>MON</td><td>TUE</td><td>WED</td><td>THU</td><td>FRI</td><td>SAT</td><td>SUN</td></tr>
</table>

SESSION:

WARM UP

CARDIOVASCULAR WORKOUT

WEIGHTS	SET 1		SET 2		SET 3		SET 4		SET 5	
EXERCISE	WEIGHT	REPS	WEIGHT	REPS	WEIGHT	REPS	WEIGHT	REPS	WEIGHT	REPS

NOTES

BREAKFAST		PROTEIN	FAT	CARBS	KCAL

LUNCH		PROTEIN	FAT	CARBS	KCAL

DINNER		PROTEIN	FAT	CARBS	KCAL

SNACKS / DRINKS		PROTEIN	FAT	CARBS	KCAL

	PROTEIN	FAT	CARBS	KCAL
DAILY TOTALS				

NOTES

DATE:		MON	TUE	WED	THU	FRI	SAT	SUN

SESSION:

WARM UP

CARDIOVASCULAR WORKOUT

WEIGHTS		SET 1		SET 2		SET 3		SET 4		SET 5	
EXERCISE		WEIGHT	REPS	WEIGHT	REPS	WEIGHT	REPS	WEIGHT	REPS	WEIGHT	REPS

NOTES

BREAKFAST	PROTEIN	FAT	CARBS	KCAL
LUNCH				
DINNER				
SNACKS / DRINKS				

	PROTEIN	FAT	CARBS	KCAL
DAILY TOTALS				

NOTES

DATE:		MON	TUE	WED	THU	FRI	SAT	SUN

SESSION:

WARM UP

CARDIOVASCULAR WORKOUT

WEIGHTS	SET 1		SET 2		SET 3		SET 4		SET 5	
EXERCISE	WEIGHT	REPS	WEIGHT	REPS	WEIGHT	REPS	WEIGHT	REPS	WEIGHT	REPS

NOTES

BREAKFAST		PROTEIN	FAT	CARBS	KCAL

LUNCH		PROTEIN	FAT	CARBS	KCAL

DINNER		PROTEIN	FAT	CARBS	KCAL

SNACKS / DRINKS		PROTEIN	FAT	CARBS	KCAL

	PROTEIN	FAT	CARBS	KCAL
DAILY TOTALS				

NOTES

DATE:			MON	TUE	WED	THU	FRI	SAT	SUN

SESSION:

WARM UP

CARDIOVASCULAR WORKOUT

WEIGHTS	SET 1		SET 2		SET 3		SET 4		SET 5	
EXERCISE	WEIGHT	REPS	WEIGHT	REPS	WEIGHT	REPS	WEIGHT	REPS	WEIGHT	REPS

NOTES

BREAKFAST		PROTEIN	FAT	CARBS	KCAL

LUNCH		PROTEIN	FAT	CARBS	KCAL

DINNER		PROTEIN	FAT	CARBS	KCAL

SNACKS / DRINKS		PROTEIN	FAT	CARBS	KCAL

	PROTEIN	FAT	CARBS	KCAL
DAILY TOTALS				

NOTES

DATE:			MON	TUE	WED	THU	FRI	SAT	SUN

SESSION:

WARM UP

CARDIOVASCULAR WORKOUT

WEIGHTS		SET 1		SET 2		SET 3		SET 4		SET 5	
EXERCISE		WEIGHT	REPS	WEIGHT	REPS	WEIGHT	REPS	WEIGHT	REPS	WEIGHT	REPS

NOTES

BREAKFAST		PROTEIN	FAT	CARBS	KCAL

LUNCH		PROTEIN	FAT	CARBS	KCAL

DINNER		PROTEIN	FAT	CARBS	KCAL

SNACKS / DRINKS		PROTEIN	FAT	CARBS	KCAL

	PROTEIN	FAT	CARBS	KCAL
DAILY TOTALS				

NOTES

DATE:		MON	TUE	WED	THU	FRI	SAT	SUN

SESSION:

WARM UP

CARDIOVASCULAR WORKOUT

WEIGHTS	SET 1		SET 2		SET 3		SET 4		SET 5	
EXERCISE	WEIGHT	REPS	WEIGHT	REPS	WEIGHT	REPS	WEIGHT	REPS	WEIGHT	REPS

NOTES

BREAKFAST	PROTEIN	FAT	CARBS	KCAL
LUNCH	PROTEIN	FAT	CARBS	KCAL
DINNER	PROTEIN	FAT	CARBS	KCAL
SNACKS / DRINKS	PROTEIN	FAT	CARBS	KCAL

	PROTEIN	FAT	CARBS	KCAL
DAILY TOTALS				

NOTES

DATE:		MON	TUE	WED	THU	FRI	SAT	SUN

SESSION:

WARM UP

CARDIOVASCULAR WORKOUT

WEIGHTS		SET 1		SET 2		SET 3		SET 4		SET 5	
EXERCISE		WEIGHT	REPS	WEIGHT	REPS	WEIGHT	REPS	WEIGHT	REPS	WEIGHT	REPS

NOTES

BREAKFAST		PROTEIN	FAT	CARBS	KCAL

LUNCH		PROTEIN	FAT	CARBS	KCAL

DINNER		PROTEIN	FAT	CARBS	KCAL

SNACKS / DRINKS		PROTEIN	FAT	CARBS	KCAL

	PROTEIN	FAT	CARBS	KCAL
DAILY TOTALS				

NOTES

DATE:		MON	TUE	WED	THU	FRI	SAT	SUN

SESSION:

WARM UP

CARDIOVASCULAR WORKOUT

WEIGHTS	SET 1		SET 2		SET 3		SET 4		SET 5	
EXERCISE	WEIGHT	REPS	WEIGHT	REPS	WEIGHT	REPS	WEIGHT	REPS	WEIGHT	REPS

NOTES

BREAKFAST	PROTEIN	FAT	CARBS	KCAL

LUNCH	PROTEIN	FAT	CARBS	KCAL

DINNER	PROTEIN	FAT	CARBS	KCAL

SNACKS / DRINKS	PROTEIN	FAT	CARBS	KCAL

	PROTEIN	FAT	CARBS	KCAL
DAILY TOTALS				

NOTES

DATE:		MON	TUE	WED	THU	FRI	SAT	SUN

SESSION:

WARM UP

CARDIOVASCULAR WORKOUT

WEIGHTS		SET 1		SET 2		SET 3		SET 4		SET 5	
EXERCISE		WEIGHT	REPS	WEIGHT	REPS	WEIGHT	REPS	WEIGHT	REPS	WEIGHT	REPS

NOTES

BREAKFAST	PROTEIN	FAT	CARBS	KCAL

LUNCH				

DINNER				

SNACKS / DRINKS				

	PROTEIN	FAT	CARBS	KCAL
DAILY TOTALS				

NOTES

DATE:			MON	TUE	WED	THU	FRI	SAT	SUN

SESSION:

WARM UP

CARDIOVASCULAR WORKOUT

WEIGHTS		SET 1		SET 2		SET 3		SET 4		SET 5	
EXERCISE	WEIGHT	REPS	WEIGHT	REPS	WEIGHT	REPS	WEIGHT	REPS	WEIGHT	REPS	

NOTES

BREAKFAST		PROTEIN	FAT	CARBS	KCAL

LUNCH					

DINNER					

SNACKS / DRINKS					

	PROTEIN	FAT	CARBS	KCAL
DAILY TOTALS				

NOTES

DATE:		MON	TUE	WED	THU	FRI	SAT	SUN

SESSION:

WARM UP

CARDIOVASCULAR WORKOUT

WEIGHTS		SET 1		SET 2		SET 3		SET 4		SET 5	
EXERCISE		WEIGHT	REPS	WEIGHT	REPS	WEIGHT	REPS	WEIGHT	REPS	WEIGHT	REPS

NOTES

BREAKFAST	PROTEIN	FAT	CARBS	KCAL

LUNCH	PROTEIN	FAT	CARBS	KCAL

DINNER	PROTEIN	FAT	CARBS	KCAL

SNACKS / DRINKS	PROTEIN	FAT	CARBS	KCAL

	PROTEIN	FAT	CARBS	KCAL
DAILY TOTALS				

NOTES

<table>
<tr><td>DATE:</td><td>MON</td><td>TUE</td><td>WED</td><td>THU</td><td>FRI</td><td>SAT</td><td>SUN</td></tr>
</table>

SESSION:

WARM UP

CARDIOVASCULAR WORKOUT

WEIGHTS	SET 1		SET 2		SET 3		SET 4		SET 5	
EXERCISE	WEIGHT	REPS	WEIGHT	REPS	WEIGHT	REPS	WEIGHT	REPS	WEIGHT	REPS

NOTES

BREAKFAST	PROTEIN	FAT	CARBS	KCAL

LUNCH	PROTEIN	FAT	CARBS	KCAL

DINNER	PROTEIN	FAT	CARBS	KCAL

SNACKS / DRINKS	PROTEIN	FAT	CARBS	KCAL

	PROTEIN	FAT	CARBS	KCAL
DAILY TOTALS				

NOTES

DATE:		MON	TUE	WED	THU	FRI	SAT	SUN

SESSION:

WARM UP

CARDIOVASCULAR WORKOUT

WEIGHTS	SET 1		SET 2		SET 3		SET 4		SET 5	
EXERCISE	WEIGHT	REPS	WEIGHT	REPS	WEIGHT	REPS	WEIGHT	REPS	WEIGHT	REPS

NOTES

BREAKFAST	PROTEIN	FAT	CARBS	KCAL

LUNCH	PROTEIN	FAT	CARBS	KCAL

DINNER	PROTEIN	FAT	CARBS	KCAL

SNACKS / DRINKS	PROTEIN	FAT	CARBS	KCAL

	PROTEIN	FAT	CARBS	KCAL
DAILY TOTALS				

NOTES

DATE:			MON	TUE	WED	THU	FRI	SAT	SUN

SESSION:

WARM UP

CARDIOVASCULAR WORKOUT

WEIGHTS		SET 1		SET 2		SET 3		SET 4		SET 5	
EXERCISE	WEIGHT	REPS	WEIGHT	REPS	WEIGHT	REPS	WEIGHT	REPS	WEIGHT	REPS

NOTES

BREAKFAST			PROTEIN	FAT	CARBS	KCAL

LUNCH						

DINNER						

SNACKS / DRINKS						

	PROTEIN	FAT	CARBS	KCAL
DAILY TOTALS				

NOTES

DATE:		MON	TUE	WED	THU	FRI	SAT	SUN

SESSION:

WARM UP

CARDIOVASCULAR WORKOUT

WEIGHTS		SET 1		SET 2		SET 3		SET 4		SET 5	
EXERCISE		WEIGHT	REPS	WEIGHT	REPS	WEIGHT	REPS	WEIGHT	REPS	WEIGHT	REPS

NOTES

<table>
<tr><td>BREAKFAST</td><td>PROTEIN</td><td>FAT</td><td>CARBS</td><td>KCAL</td></tr>
<tr><td></td><td></td><td></td><td></td><td></td></tr>
<tr><td></td><td></td><td></td><td></td><td></td></tr>
<tr><td></td><td></td><td></td><td></td><td></td></tr>
<tr><td></td><td></td><td></td><td></td><td></td></tr>
</table>

<table>
<tr><td>LUNCH</td><td></td><td></td><td></td><td></td></tr>
<tr><td></td><td></td><td></td><td></td><td></td></tr>
<tr><td></td><td></td><td></td><td></td><td></td></tr>
<tr><td></td><td></td><td></td><td></td><td></td></tr>
<tr><td></td><td></td><td></td><td></td><td></td></tr>
</table>

<table>
<tr><td>DINNER</td><td></td><td></td><td></td><td></td></tr>
<tr><td></td><td></td><td></td><td></td><td></td></tr>
<tr><td></td><td></td><td></td><td></td><td></td></tr>
<tr><td></td><td></td><td></td><td></td><td></td></tr>
<tr><td></td><td></td><td></td><td></td><td></td></tr>
</table>

<table>
<tr><td>SNACKS / DRINKS</td><td></td><td></td><td></td><td></td></tr>
<tr><td></td><td></td><td></td><td></td><td></td></tr>
<tr><td></td><td></td><td></td><td></td><td></td></tr>
<tr><td></td><td></td><td></td><td></td><td></td></tr>
<tr><td></td><td></td><td></td><td></td><td></td></tr>
</table>

	PROTEIN	FAT	CARBS	KCAL
DAILY TOTALS				

NOTES

DATE:		MON	TUE	WED	THU	FRI	SAT	SUN

SESSION:

WARM UP

CARDIOVASCULAR WORKOUT

WEIGHTS	SET 1		SET 2		SET 3		SET 4		SET 5	
EXERCISE	WEIGHT	REPS	WEIGHT	REPS	WEIGHT	REPS	WEIGHT	REPS	WEIGHT	REPS

NOTES

BREAKFAST	PROTEIN	FAT	CARBS	KCAL

LUNCH	PROTEIN	FAT	CARBS	KCAL

DINNER	PROTEIN	FAT	CARBS	KCAL

SNACKS / DRINKS	PROTEIN	FAT	CARBS	KCAL

	PROTEIN	FAT	CARBS	KCAL
DAILY TOTALS				

NOTES

DATE:			MON	TUE	WED	THU	FRI	SAT	SUN

SESSION:

WARM UP

CARDIOVASCULAR WORKOUT

WEIGHTS		SET 1		SET 2		SET 3		SET 4		SET 5	
EXERCISE		WEIGHT	REPS	WEIGHT	REPS	WEIGHT	REPS	WEIGHT	REPS	WEIGHT	REPS

NOTES

BREAKFAST		PROTEIN	FAT	CARBS	KCAL

LUNCH		PROTEIN	FAT	CARBS	KCAL

DINNER		PROTEIN	FAT	CARBS	KCAL

SNACKS / DRINKS		PROTEIN	FAT	CARBS	KCAL

	PROTEIN	FAT	CARBS	KCAL
DAILY TOTALS				

NOTES

DATE:		MON	TUE	WED	THU	FRI	SAT	SUN

SESSION:

WARM UP

CARDIOVASCULAR WORKOUT

WEIGHTS		SET 1		SET 2		SET 3		SET 4		SET 5	
EXERCISE	WEIGHT	REPS	WEIGHT	REPS	WEIGHT	REPS	WEIGHT	REPS	WEIGHT	REPS

NOTES

BREAKFAST		PROTEIN	FAT	CARBS	KCAL

LUNCH		PROTEIN	FAT	CARBS	KCAL

DINNER		PROTEIN	FAT	CARBS	KCAL

SNACKS / DRINKS		PROTEIN	FAT	CARBS	KCAL

	PROTEIN	FAT	CARBS	KCAL
DAILY TOTALS				

NOTES

DATE:		MON	TUE	WED	THU	FRI	SAT	SUN

SESSION:

WARM UP

CARDIOVASCULAR WORKOUT

WEIGHTS	SET 1		SET 2		SET 3		SET 4		SET 5	
EXERCISE	WEIGHT	REPS	WEIGHT	REPS	WEIGHT	REPS	WEIGHT	REPS	WEIGHT	REPS

NOTES

BREAKFAST		PROTEIN	FAT	CARBS	KCAL

LUNCH					

DINNER					

SNACKS / DRINKS					

	PROTEIN	FAT	CARBS	KCAL
DAILY TOTALS				

NOTES

DATE:		MON	TUE	WED	THU	FRI	SAT	SUN

SESSION:

WARM UP

CARDIOVASCULAR WORKOUT

WEIGHTS		SET 1		SET 2		SET 3		SET 4		SET 5	
EXERCISE		WEIGHT	REPS	WEIGHT	REPS	WEIGHT	REPS	WEIGHT	REPS	WEIGHT	REPS

NOTES

BREAKFAST	PROTEIN	FAT	CARBS	KCAL

LUNCH	PROTEIN	FAT	CARBS	KCAL

DINNER	PROTEIN	FAT	CARBS	KCAL

SNACKS / DRINKS	PROTEIN	FAT	CARBS	KCAL

	PROTEIN	FAT	CARBS	KCAL
DAILY TOTALS				

NOTES

DATE:		MON	TUE	WED	THU	FRI	SAT	SUN

SESSION:

WARM UP

CARDIOVASCULAR WORKOUT

WEIGHTS		SET 1		SET 2		SET 3		SET 4		SET 5	
EXERCISE		WEIGHT	REPS	WEIGHT	REPS	WEIGHT	REPS	WEIGHT	REPS	WEIGHT	REPS

NOTES

BREAKFAST		PROTEIN	FAT	CARBS	KCAL

LUNCH					

DINNER					

SNACKS / DRINKS					

	PROTEIN	FAT	CARBS	KCAL
DAILY TOTALS				

NOTES

DATE:			MON	TUE	WED	THU	FRI	SAT	SUN

SESSION:

WARM UP

CARDIOVASCULAR WORKOUT

WEIGHTS	SET 1		SET 2		SET 3		SET 4		SET 5	
EXERCISE	WEIGHT	REPS	WEIGHT	REPS	WEIGHT	REPS	WEIGHT	REPS	WEIGHT	REPS

NOTES

BREAKFAST			PROTEIN	FAT	CARBS	KCAL

LUNCH						

DINNER						

SNACKS / DRINKS						

	PROTEIN	FAT	CARBS	KCAL
DAILY TOTALS				

NOTES

DATE:		MON	TUE	WED	THU	FRI	SAT	SUN

SESSION:

WARM UP

CARDIOVASCULAR WORKOUT

WEIGHTS	SET 1		SET 2		SET 3		SET 4		SET 5	
EXERCISE	WEIGHT	REPS	WEIGHT	REPS	WEIGHT	REPS	WEIGHT	REPS	WEIGHT	REPS

NOTES

BREAKFAST		PROTEIN	FAT	CARBS	KCAL
LUNCH					
DINNER					
SNACKS / DRINKS					

	PROTEIN	FAT	CARBS	KCAL
DAILY TOTALS				

NOTES

DATE:		MON	TUE	WED	THU	FRI	SAT	SUN

SESSION:

WARM UP

CARDIOVASCULAR WORKOUT

WEIGHTS	SET 1		SET 2		SET 3		SET 4		SET 5	
EXERCISE	WEIGHT	REPS	WEIGHT	REPS	WEIGHT	REPS	WEIGHT	REPS	WEIGHT	REPS

NOTES

BREAKFAST		PROTEIN	FAT	CARBS	KCAL

LUNCH		PROTEIN	FAT	CARBS	KCAL

DINNER		PROTEIN	FAT	CARBS	KCAL

SNACKS / DRINKS		PROTEIN	FAT	CARBS	KCAL

	PROTEIN	FAT	CARBS	KCAL
DAILY TOTALS				

NOTES

DATE:		MON	TUE	WED	THU	FRI	SAT	SUN

SESSION:

WARM UP

CARDIOVASCULAR WORKOUT

WEIGHTS	SET 1		SET 2		SET 3		SET 4		SET 5	
EXERCISE	WEIGHT	REPS	WEIGHT	REPS	WEIGHT	REPS	WEIGHT	REPS	WEIGHT	REPS

NOTES

BREAKFAST		PROTEIN	FAT	CARBS	KCAL

LUNCH					

DINNER					

SNACKS / DRINKS					

	PROTEIN	FAT	CARBS	KCAL
DAILY TOTALS				

NOTES

DATE:		MON	TUE	WED	THU	FRI	SAT	SUN

SESSION:

WARM UP

CARDIOVASCULAR WORKOUT

WEIGHTS	SET 1		SET 2		SET 3		SET 4		SET 5	
EXERCISE	WEIGHT	REPS	WEIGHT	REPS	WEIGHT	REPS	WEIGHT	REPS	WEIGHT	REPS

NOTES

BREAKFAST		PROTEIN	FAT	CARBS	KCAL

LUNCH					

DINNER					

SNACKS / DRINKS					

	PROTEIN	FAT	CARBS	KCAL
DAILY TOTALS				

NOTES

DATE:		MON	TUE	WED	THU	FRI	SAT	SUN

SESSION:

WARM UP

CARDIOVASCULAR WORKOUT

WEIGHTS		SET 1		SET 2		SET 3		SET 4		SET 5	
EXERCISE		WEIGHT	REPS	WEIGHT	REPS	WEIGHT	REPS	WEIGHT	REPS	WEIGHT	REPS

NOTES

BREAKFAST		PROTEIN	FAT	CARBS	KCAL

LUNCH		PROTEIN	FAT	CARBS	KCAL

DINNER		PROTEIN	FAT	CARBS	KCAL

SNACKS / DRINKS		PROTEIN	FAT	CARBS	KCAL

	PROTEIN	FAT	CARBS	KCAL
DAILY TOTALS				

NOTES

DATE:			MON	TUE	WED	THU	FRI	SAT	SUN

SESSION:

WARM UP

CARDIOVASCULAR WORKOUT

WEIGHTS	SET 1		SET 2		SET 3		SET 4		SET 5	
EXERCISE	WEIGHT	REPS	WEIGHT	REPS	WEIGHT	REPS	WEIGHT	REPS	WEIGHT	REPS

NOTES

BREAKFAST	PROTEIN	FAT	CARBS	KCAL

LUNCH				

DINNER				

SNACKS / DRINKS				

	PROTEIN	FAT	CARBS	KCAL
DAILY TOTALS				

NOTES

DATE:		MON	TUE	WED	THU	FRI	SAT	SUN

SESSION:

WARM UP

CARDIOVASCULAR WORKOUT

WEIGHTS	SET 1		SET 2		SET 3		SET 4		SET 5	
EXERCISE	WEIGHT	REPS	WEIGHT	REPS	WEIGHT	REPS	WEIGHT	REPS	WEIGHT	REPS

NOTES

BREAKFAST		PROTEIN	FAT	CARBS	KCAL

LUNCH		PROTEIN	FAT	CARBS	KCAL

DINNER		PROTEIN	FAT	CARBS	KCAL

SNACKS / DRINKS		PROTEIN	FAT	CARBS	KCAL

	PROTEIN	FAT	CARBS	KCAL
DAILY TOTALS				

NOTES

DATE:		MON	TUE	WED	THU	FRI	SAT	SUN

SESSION:

WARM UP

CARDIOVASCULAR WORKOUT

WEIGHTS		SET 1		SET 2		SET 3		SET 4		SET 5	
EXERCISE	WEIGHT	REPS	WEIGHT	REPS	WEIGHT	REPS	WEIGHT	REPS	WEIGHT	REPS

NOTES

BREAKFAST		PROTEIN	FAT	CARBS	KCAL
LUNCH					
DINNER					
SNACKS / DRINKS					

	PROTEIN	FAT	CARBS	KCAL
DAILY TOTALS				

NOTES

DATE:		MON	TUE	WED	THU	FRI	SAT	SUN

SESSION:

WARM UP

CARDIOVASCULAR WORKOUT

WEIGHTS		SET 1		SET 2		SET 3		SET 4		SET 5	
EXERCISE		WEIGHT	REPS	WEIGHT	REPS	WEIGHT	REPS	WEIGHT	REPS	WEIGHT	REPS

NOTES

BREAKFAST		PROTEIN	FAT	CARBS	KCAL

LUNCH		PROTEIN	FAT	CARBS	KCAL

DINNER		PROTEIN	FAT	CARBS	KCAL

SNACKS / DRINKS		PROTEIN	FAT	CARBS	KCAL

	PROTEIN	FAT	CARBS	KCAL
DAILY TOTALS				

NOTES

DATE:		MON	TUE	WED	THU	FRI	SAT	SUN

SESSION:

WARM UP

CARDIOVASCULAR WORKOUT

WEIGHTS		SET 1		SET 2		SET 3		SET 4		SET 5	
EXERCISE		WEIGHT	REPS	WEIGHT	REPS	WEIGHT	REPS	WEIGHT	REPS	WEIGHT	REPS

NOTES

BREAKFAST	PROTEIN	FAT	CARBS	KCAL

LUNCH	PROTEIN	FAT	CARBS	KCAL

DINNER	PROTEIN	FAT	CARBS	KCAL

SNACKS / DRINKS	PROTEIN	FAT	CARBS	KCAL

	PROTEIN	FAT	CARBS	KCAL
DAILY TOTALS				

NOTES

DATE:		MON	TUE	WED	THU	FRI	SAT	SUN

SESSION:

WARM UP

CARDIOVASCULAR WORKOUT

WEIGHTS		SET 1		SET 2		SET 3		SET 4		SET 5	
EXERCISE	WEIGHT	REPS	WEIGHT	REPS	WEIGHT	REPS	WEIGHT	REPS	WEIGHT	REPS	

NOTES

BREAKFAST		PROTEIN	FAT	CARBS	KCAL

LUNCH		PROTEIN	FAT	CARBS	KCAL

DINNER		PROTEIN	FAT	CARBS	KCAL

SNACKS / DRINKS		PROTEIN	FAT	CARBS	KCAL

	PROTEIN	FAT	CARBS	KCAL
DAILY TOTALS				

NOTES

DATE:			MON	TUE	WED	THU	FRI	SAT	SUN

SESSION:

WARM UP

CARDIOVASCULAR WORKOUT

WEIGHTS		SET 1		SET 2		SET 3		SET 4		SET 5	
EXERCISE	WEIGHT	REPS	WEIGHT	REPS	WEIGHT	REPS	WEIGHT	REPS	WEIGHT	REPS

NOTES

BREAKFAST	PROTEIN	FAT	CARBS	KCAL

LUNCH	PROTEIN	FAT	CARBS	KCAL

DINNER	PROTEIN	FAT	CARBS	KCAL

SNACKS / DRINKS	PROTEIN	FAT	CARBS	KCAL

	PROTEIN	FAT	CARBS	KCAL
DAILY TOTALS				

NOTES

DATE:		MON	TUE	WED	THU	FRI	SAT	SUN

SESSION:

WARM UP

CARDIOVASCULAR WORKOUT

WEIGHTS	SET 1		SET 2		SET 3		SET 4		SET 5	
EXERCISE	WEIGHT	REPS	WEIGHT	REPS	WEIGHT	REPS	WEIGHT	REPS	WEIGHT	REPS

NOTES

BREAKFAST		PROTEIN	FAT	CARBS	KCAL

LUNCH		PROTEIN	FAT	CARBS	KCAL

DINNER		PROTEIN	FAT	CARBS	KCAL

SNACKS / DRINKS		PROTEIN	FAT	CARBS	KCAL

	PROTEIN	FAT	CARBS	KCAL
DAILY TOTALS				

NOTES

DATE:			MON	TUE	WED	THU	FRI	SAT	SUN

SESSION:

WARM UP

CARDIOVASCULAR WORKOUT

WEIGHTS		SET 1		SET 2		SET 3		SET 4		SET 5	
EXERCISE		WEIGHT	REPS	WEIGHT	REPS	WEIGHT	REPS	WEIGHT	REPS	WEIGHT	REPS

NOTES

BREAKFAST	PROTEIN	FAT	CARBS	KCAL

LUNCH	PROTEIN	FAT	CARBS	KCAL

DINNER	PROTEIN	FAT	CARBS	KCAL

SNACKS / DRINKS	PROTEIN	FAT	CARBS	KCAL

	PROTEIN	FAT	CARBS	KCAL
DAILY TOTALS				

NOTES

DATE:		MON	TUE	WED	THU	FRI	SAT	SUN

SESSION:

WARM UP

CARDIOVASCULAR WORKOUT

WEIGHTS	SET 1		SET 2		SET 3		SET 4		SET 5	
EXERCISE	WEIGHT	REPS	WEIGHT	REPS	WEIGHT	REPS	WEIGHT	REPS	WEIGHT	REPS

NOTES

BREAKFAST		PROTEIN	FAT	CARBS	KCAL

LUNCH		PROTEIN	FAT	CARBS	KCAL

DINNER		PROTEIN	FAT	CARBS	KCAL

SNACKS / DRINKS		PROTEIN	FAT	CARBS	KCAL

	PROTEIN	FAT	CARBS	KCAL
DAILY TOTALS				

NOTES

<table>
<tr><td>DATE:</td><td>MON</td><td>TUE</td><td>WED</td><td>THU</td><td>FRI</td><td>SAT</td><td>SUN</td></tr>
</table>

SESSION:

WARM UP

CARDIOVASCULAR WORKOUT

WEIGHTS	SET 1		SET 2		SET 3		SET 4		SET 5	
EXERCISE	WEIGHT	REPS	WEIGHT	REPS	WEIGHT	REPS	WEIGHT	REPS	WEIGHT	REPS

NOTES

<table>
<tr><td>BREAKFAST</td><td>PROTEIN</td><td>FAT</td><td>CARBS</td><td>KCAL</td></tr>
</table>

<table>
<tr><td>LUNCH</td><td></td><td></td><td></td><td></td></tr>
</table>

<table>
<tr><td>DINNER</td><td></td><td></td><td></td><td></td></tr>
</table>

<table>
<tr><td>SNACKS / DRINKS</td><td></td><td></td><td></td><td></td></tr>
</table>

	PROTEIN	FAT	CARBS	KCAL
DAILY TOTALS				

NOTES

DATE:			MON	TUE	WED	THU	FRI	SAT	SUN

SESSION:

WARM UP

CARDIOVASCULAR WORKOUT

WEIGHTS		SET 1		SET 2		SET 3		SET 4		SET 5	
EXERCISE	WEIGHT	REPS	WEIGHT	REPS	WEIGHT	REPS	WEIGHT	REPS	WEIGHT	REPS

NOTES

BREAKFAST		PROTEIN	FAT	CARBS	KCAL
LUNCH					
DINNER					
SNACKS / DRINKS					

	PROTEIN	FAT	CARBS	KCAL
DAILY TOTALS				

NOTES

DATE:		MON	TUE	WED	THU	FRI	SAT	SUN

SESSION:

WARM UP

CARDIOVASCULAR WORKOUT

WEIGHTS		SET 1		SET 2		SET 3		SET 4		SET 5	
EXERCISE		WEIGHT	REPS	WEIGHT	REPS	WEIGHT	REPS	WEIGHT	REPS	WEIGHT	REPS

NOTES

BREAKFAST	PROTEIN	FAT	CARBS	KCAL

LUNCH	PROTEIN	FAT	CARBS	KCAL

DINNER	PROTEIN	FAT	CARBS	KCAL

SNACKS / DRINKS	PROTEIN	FAT	CARBS	KCAL

	PROTEIN	FAT	CARBS	KCAL
DAILY TOTALS				

NOTES

DATE:		MON	TUE	WED	THU	FRI	SAT	SUN

SESSION:

WARM UP

CARDIOVASCULAR WORKOUT

WEIGHTS	SET 1		SET 2		SET 3		SET 4		SET 5	
EXERCISE	WEIGHT	REPS	WEIGHT	REPS	WEIGHT	REPS	WEIGHT	REPS	WEIGHT	REPS

NOTES

BREAKFAST	PROTEIN	FAT	CARBS	KCAL

LUNCH	PROTEIN	FAT	CARBS	KCAL

DINNER	PROTEIN	FAT	CARBS	KCAL

SNACKS / DRINKS	PROTEIN	FAT	CARBS	KCAL

	PROTEIN	FAT	CARBS	KCAL
DAILY TOTALS				

NOTES

DATE:			MON	TUE	WED	THU	FRI	SAT	SUN

SESSION:

WARM UP

CARDIOVASCULAR WORKOUT

WEIGHTS		SET 1		SET 2		SET 3		SET 4		SET 5	
EXERCISE	WEIGHT	REPS	WEIGHT	REPS	WEIGHT	REPS	WEIGHT	REPS	WEIGHT	REPS

NOTES

BREAKFAST		PROTEIN	FAT	CARBS	KCAL

LUNCH					

DINNER					

SNACKS / DRINKS					

	PROTEIN	FAT	CARBS	KCAL
DAILY TOTALS				

NOTES